My Health

My Right

THE COMPLETE HEALTH GUIDE

By

Prakash . M

DISCLAIMER AND TERMS OF USE AGREEMENT

Introduction

Health is the ability of a biological system to acquire, convert, allocate, distribute, and utilize energy with maximum efficiency.

The World Health Organization describes mental health as "a state of well-being in which the individual realizes his or her own abilities, can cope with the normal stresses of life, can work productively and fruitfully, and is able to make a contribution to his or her community

Now the word health is becoming a business item! Read this book well. Understand about the body and inner organs activities. Think about the truths revealed in this book about the body. Then practice the habits suggested in this book. This book suggest to change many of your habits.

At the beginning it is difficult to follow the all habits. But start with few things, then try to change your all habits. If you have disease, it will cure. Your immunity power will increase. Why do you fear? Let's see in detail in this book about something vital to life.

Let's see in detail about how to live in our everyday life without using drugs and other things. This is the basic guide to being in everyone's hands. These are the methods are followed by the millions of people in olden days and also in now a days also.

The modern medical world gives only quick relief for all, but not full complete cure of any disease. If you follow these methods it will give permanent cure but it will take some time.

This book reveals the power of the body, which have the ability to heal anything defected in our body. That means self-treatment to yourself. And also you can understand " disease are not appeared in one day and it is the series of small defects created day by day in our body.

HEALTH

Health is the ability of a biological system to acquire, convert, allocate, distribute, and utilize energy with maximum efficiency. Your human body should work with full efficiency until the end of life. All of your physical body and internal organs should be work perfectly.

What we have to do..?

First you should understand what are the factors that affecting your human body.

1. Your mental health
2. Air that you breathe
3. Water which you consume
4. Food which you take
5. Environmental conditions
6. Your habits

If you organize the six of the above, you will be healthy throughout life.

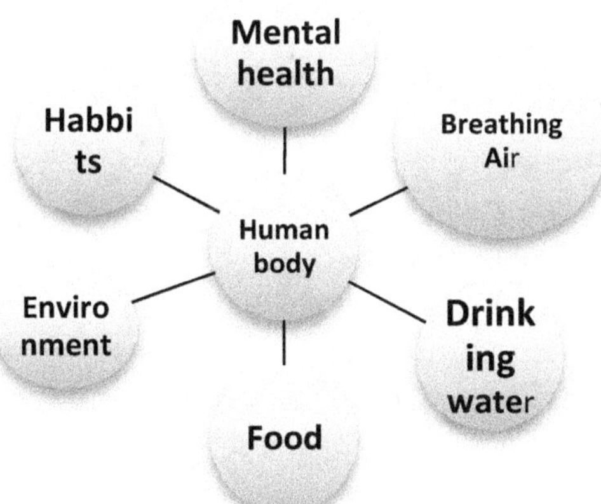

1. Your mental health

There is a direct connection to the mind and body. When we think of some favorite foods, our body will sprinkle the saliva. The mind is linked to the body and the saliva is secreted. Similarly, the mind controls or interferes with all body organs. For example During the feelings of fear, it increases the speed of breathing. When we meditate , the breathing speed decreases.

The function of the internal organs of the body is controlled by the subconscious mind.

So it is very important to maintain the mental health to be healthy.

The factors affecting the Mind

1. Work
2. Environment,
3. People around you and their speech
4. Worry
5. Fear and so on

Some ways to keep your mind well

1. Choose your favorite job
2. Be grateful
3. Be friendly to everyone.
4. Do breathing exercise every day or meditate.

Simple meditation

1. In a well-ventilated, quiet room or outdoor, sit in the Yoga mat, or sit in the chair.
2. Close your eyes and watch your breath inhale and exhale.
3.Do this daily 20 minutes.
4.After the meditation , rub your hands with your hands gently and open your eyes slowly and see your palms.

Benefits of Meditation

1. Depression decreases and stress reduces.
2. It gives peace of mind.
3. This lead to good thinking.
4. Your body also get benefit from this.

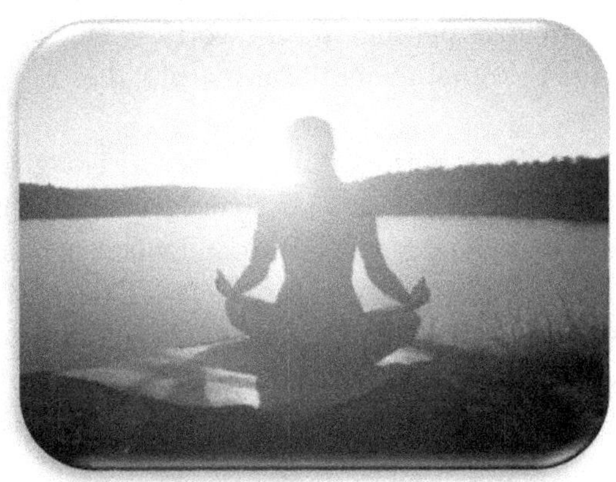

Breathing Exercise

1. In a well-ventilated, quiet room or out door, sit in the Yoga mat, or sit in the chair.
2. Close your eyes and inhale your breath in 1 sec hold it for 2 sec and exhale it for 3 second.
3.Do this daily up to 20 minutes.
4. After the Breathing exercise rub your hands with your hands gently and open your eyes slowly and see your palms.

Benefits of Breathing exercise

1. The body needs Oxygen.
2. All the nerves of the body are strengthened.
3. It gives peace of mind.

It's better than going to the hospital and waiting for the doctor. Do not leave this habbit after a day or a month. You can't get immediate benefit. But permanent benefit is there and immunity power will increase. Total body movements will improve. These habits have the ability to heal certain diseases. But these are the things you need to follow in your daily life .

2. Air

It is said that food is medicine. But, food alone cannot be medicine. We eat food for about three times in a day. But we breathe air for all the 24 hours in a day. We breathe about 11,600 litres of air in a day at the rate of 8 litres per minute. We worry so much about the food we eat but we never bother about the air we breathe.

A person inhales 8 litres of air in a minute and gives it to his lungs. The lung takes oxygen, nitrogen, hydrogen, pranic energy and many other such ingredients from the air and mixes them in the blood. These good ingredients are given to the cells in all the parts of the body through the blood. Each cell takes the energy from these ingredients, converts them into bad ingredients and this waste(carbon di oxide) matter comes back to the blood.

Human Gas Exchange Process

When the waste matter in the blood comes to the lung, the lung sends it out through the nose in the air we breathe out. So, whenever we breathe, we inhale good air and exhale bad air. If four persons sleep in a room, at the rate of 8 litres per minute per person, these four persons convert all the air in that room into bad air in about half an hour. We sleep for about 8 hours every night.

Good air will go into our body only for the first half an hour. Only the bad air sent out by our body will again and again go into our body for the remaining seven and a half hours. In this way, when our body does not get the air energy and all the other nutrients from the air, all our body
parts get diseases. If we sleep and breathe the bad air for seven and a half hours, how can we get good health? No one seems to think about this at all.

Now we have understood that our body will get diseases if we close all the doors and windows and sleep in a room without any air ventilation. If diseases can come even when we just sleep in a closed room, we will get even bigger diseases if we use mosquito coils, mosquito mats, etc. in a closed room and sleep in that room. we spend our own money to buy mosquito coil and we give poison to ourselves. So don't use mosquito coils, Instead of this you can use insect nets.

Remedies

- We should not use mosquito coil, mosquito repellent liquid, mosquito mat, etc.
- There should be good air ventilation at all places such as our home, office, factory,
  bed room, etc, at all times.
- We should not keep all the windows closed in our bed room when we sleep.
- We can use mosquito net to avoid mosquitoes biting us.

- Air ventilation in the places where we live should be such that good air can come in
and bad air can go out for all the 24 hours of the day.

3. Drinking Water

Water is very important for your body. This earth is a marvel of nature. There is no water anywhere in this universe except earth. In earth also 96.5 percent sea water. It is not suitable for drinking. The rest of the water in the world for is suitable for drinking. This is a rare creation.

Water on Earth

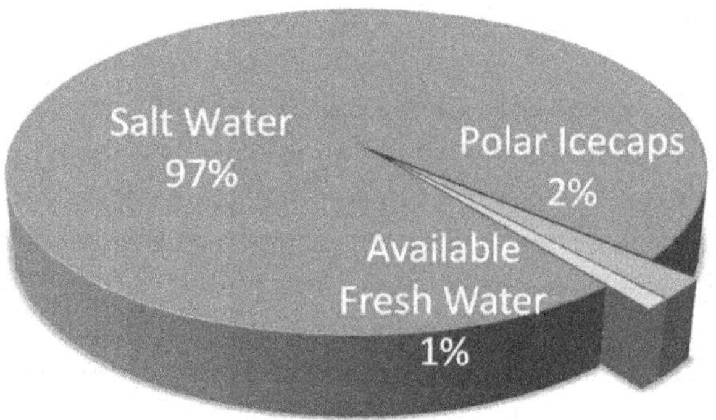

Should we boil the water ?

Why should we boil the water? We boil the water for the sole reason that there are disease-causing germs in the water and these germs get killed when the water is boiled. All right, how many litres of water do we drink daily? It may be two or three litres.

How many disease-causing germs could be there in these three litres of water? But, we inhale 11600 litres of air every day, at the rate of 8 liters per minute, through our nose. Can anyone say that there are no disease causing germs in the air? All the dust, dirt, garbage, bacteria and viruses go inside our body through the air that we breathe.

They say that disease-causing germs are there in the three litres of water that we drink daily and diseases can come due to these germs. We inhale 11600 litres of air every day. Will we not get diseases through this air?

The water we drink contains a pranic energy called Water Energy. This cannot be seen by the eyes. Moreover, many minerals and vitamins are present in the drinking water. These are essentially needed for our body. Drinking water contains nutrients, life energy as well as disease-causing germs.

People all over the world are being advised to eat organically produced fruits and vegetables. However, the fact that water will be devoid of all the organic compounds when it is boiled is not conveyed to the people by any of the health care organizations.

During the outbreak of life-threatening epidemics in the country and during Tsunami, floods, etc. all the water resources in the country would be polluted. During such times, even cattle may be lying dead in the water resources and the water may also be muddy. Sometimes, even human bodies may be lying in the water.

In those situations, we should boil the water, cool it, filter it and then only drink it. This procedure is therefore valid only during such emergency periods. Otherwise, during normal periods, there is no necessity to boil the water available in the areas where we live.

The advice that we should boil the water, cool it, filter it and drink it was propagated during emergency times because of the fact that diseases could be caused if we drink dirty and polluted water. If we follow this advice daily during normal times thinking that it is always valid, then it will cause diseases in our body.

RO and Mineral Water

We should not drink water sold in the so-called mineral water bottles. There is a machine called Anti Scale Dosing Machine in mineral water manufacturing factories. This machine removes all minerals from the water and makes it stale water.

In this way, good water is converted into stale, useless water by many processing activities and it is packaged in bottles and sold. We spend money to buy it and drink it. Therefore, please do not use the packaged drinking water called Mineral water which is devoid of any minerals.

Even though filtered water and mineral water will not have any nutrients essential for the body, they will have some Life Energy. However, boiled water will not have any Life Energy. Therefore, filtered water and mineral water are acceptable for consumption to some extent but boiled water is unacceptable at any cost.

Water should not be boiled. It should not be filtered. We should not use water packed in bottles. Then how else can we clean the water? We can drink the water that comes from the water tap as it is. There is no necessity to clean it. Ordinary tap water is the biggest and the best vaccine in the whole world.

All those who drink tap water directly will never get any disease from any germ. They will have very high immunity in their body
to fight diseases. Their body will be healthy. Therefore, please drink ordinary tap water as it comes.

If you feel that the tap water coming to your house is contaminated, for your mental satisfaction you can do a few things. You can try to purify the water in a natural way through one of the following methods.

Clay pot as Water Filter

If we pour drinking water in a mud pot and keep it for about two to five hours, the mud pot will absorb all the bad elements from the water and give Earth Energy to that water. Mud pot is the best water filter in the whole world. You have spent a good amount of money and installed a water filter in your house.

How many mud pots can you get for that money? Even if you break one pot every day, the stock will never be exhausted. But, nowadays nobody uses such a wonderful, natural water filter. So, please keep water in a mud pot and drink it. All the bad elements in the water will be destroyed. You will get Earth Energy. Your pranic energy also will increase.

White Cotton Cloth as Water Filter

If we filter the water using whitecolored clean cotton cloth then this cloth filters all the disease-causing virus, bacteria, etc. from the water. This fact has been scientifically proven. This is the reason why our forefathers did not use any medicine or tablets and did not go to any hospital when children had diseases such as measles. They cured the disease just by bathing the child in water filtered in a white cotton cloth. So, if needed, we can clean the water using this method.

We Can Clean The Water Using A Banana Skin

If we put an ordinary banana skin inside the water in a mud pot and take it out after half an hour, the banana skin absorbs all the germs and bad elements from the water in the mud pot.

But if we keep the banana skin inside the water. For a longer period, it will become garbage. So, we have to remove the banana skin within half an hour. We can use this simple method to purify the water

We can clean the water using a copper coin or a copper vessel

If we keep the water in a vessel made of copper for two to five hours, the water gets more energy. The bad elements in the water are destroyed. So, we can use vessels made of copper for storing water. If we put some copper coins inside the water in a mud pot, the copper coins will keep on purifying the water.

Do's

- When we feel thirst , we should immediately drink sufficient quantity of water to quench our thirst.
- We can keep water in an earthen pot for two hours and then use it.
- We should drink water immediately after we pass urine.
- We should drink water by slowly sipping it little by little.
- We can filter the water using a cotton cloth and then drink it.
- We can put a banana skin, copper coin or copper plate inside the water for half an hour and then drink the water.

- We should not use mineral water sold in bottles.
- We should not filter the water using water filter or water purifier.
- We should not drink water when we are not feeling thirsty.
- We should not drink water pouring it into our mouth from above.
- We should clean our drinking water tank frequently.
- There is no prescribed quantity of water that we have to compulsorily drink every day.

4 .FOOD

FIVE TYPES OF FOOD

There are several types of food. To understand them easily we have classified them into five broad types. These are

(1) fruits and natural foods,
(2) sprouted grains,
(3) cooked foods,
(4) non-vegetarian foods
(5) intoxicants and narcotics.

Let us now see in detail about these food types.

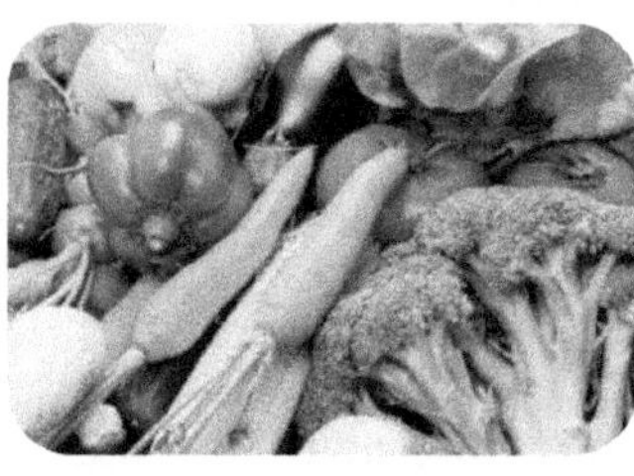

Organic
Vegetables

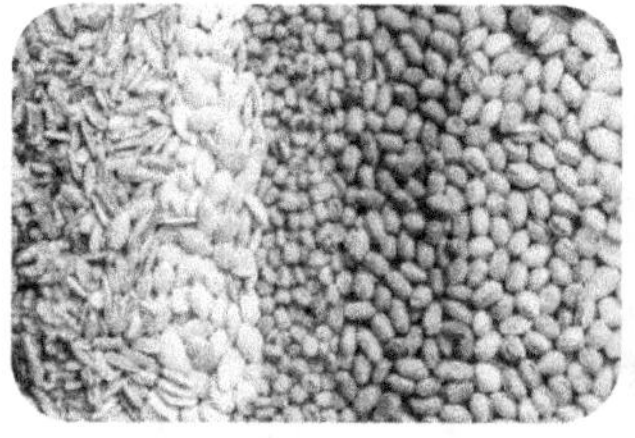

Grains

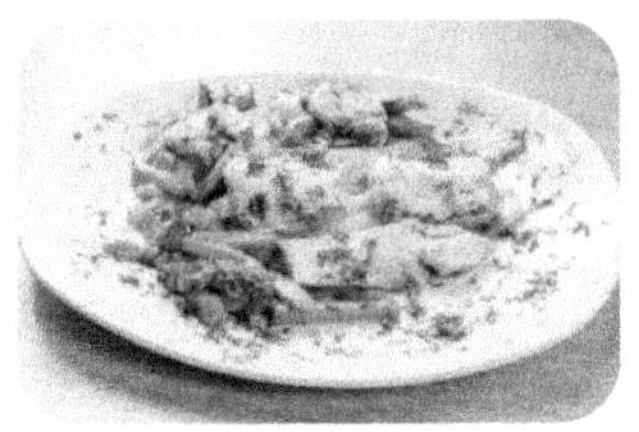

Cooked Food

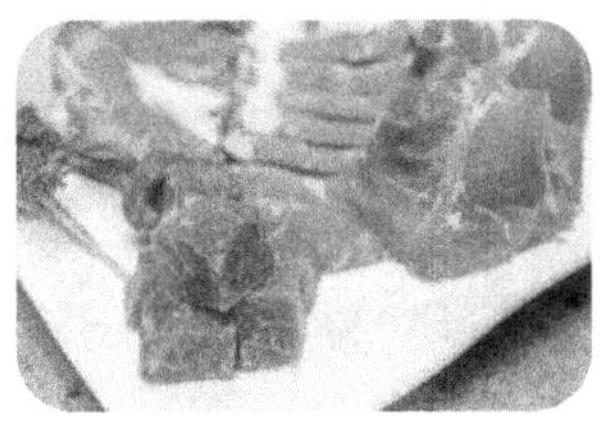

Non-veg

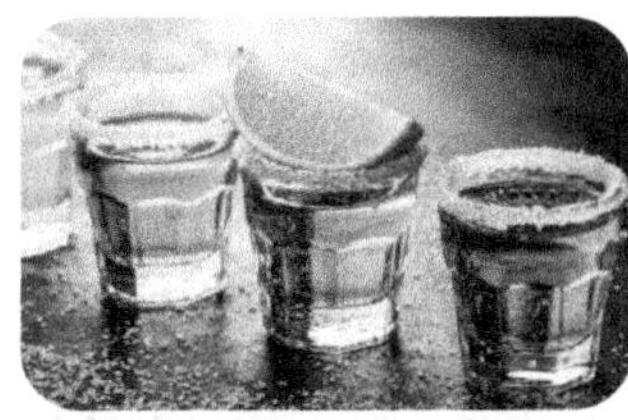

Liquor

(1)   Fruits and natural foods

The first type of food consists of all foods which are natural and tasty. All uncooked foods such as fruits, coconut, cucumber, carrot, etc, which are uncooked but at the same time are tasty belong to this group. These foods have 100% taste. So they get 100 marks for taste. These have 100% pranic energy. So they get another 100 marks for pranic energy. These have 100% nutrients. So they get another 100 marks for nutrients. So, totally the first type of food gets 300 marks. All the foods which can be eaten uncooked and raw but are also tasty come under this group.

(2)   *grains*,

The second type consists of all uncooked but not-so-tasty foods. For example, all sprouted grains and pulses, all tasteless fruits and vegetables belong to this group. This type of foods contains 100% pranic energy. So, they get 100 marks for pranic energy. These contain 100 %
nutrients. So they get 100 marks for nutrients. But these do not have taste. So, they get 0 marks for taste. So, these foods get total 200 marks. These are grouped as second type.

(3)   Cooked foods

All cooked vegetables, spinach leaves, grains, etc. belong to this third type. When we cook a food, the taste in the food reduces by 50%. So, these foods get 50 marks for taste. Also, when a food is cooked, it loses 50% of its nutrients. So these foodsget 50 marks for nutrients. Also these foods lose 50% of their pranic energy when cooked. So, these foods get 50 marks for pranic energy. So totally this type of food gets 150 marks. All cooked dishes that we normally eat come under this group.

(4)   Non-Vegetarian

The non-vegetarian foods come under this fourth category. Non-veg foods contain 100% nutrients. So, they get 100 marks for nutrients. There will be no pranic energy in them. So, they get no marks for pranic energy. There will be no taste in them. So, they get no marks for taste. So, non-veg. foods get a total of 100 marks. Therefore, it is good to avoid or reduce non-veg. foods as far as possible.

But, in some desert areas and hot countries, due to the non availability of plant foods, there may be a necessity to eat non veg. foods. Anatomically, nothing wrong will happen to our body if we eat non-veg. food.

But, on spiritual grounds, if our mind has developed a thought that it is a sin to kill a living being, when we eat non-veg. food, that thought will create disease in our body.

So, when non-veg. eaters eat the non veg. food with the thought that eating it is not a sin and eat it without any confusion in their mind, then the food gets digested properly. If they eat it with the dilemma "Is it right or wrong to eat it?" then that thought creates diseases in the body. This is not only true for non-veg. foods. This is true for all foods. If we eat any food with the clear and strong conviction and belief that it is good for our health, then that food acts as medicine. If we eat it with the doubtful thought that it might create disease in our body, it actually creates diseases. Finally, it is advisable to avoid non vegetarian foods.

All the narcotic drugs belong to this group. These are actually not foods. We consume some narcotics and intoxicants as if they are food items. But those items are not foods. All intoxicants such as tea, coffee, cigarette, liquor, Paan, ganja, areca nut, etc. belong to this category. How to know the difference between intoxicants and food items? All those items by eating which, thrice daily, we can remain alive are food items. If we cannot remain alive just by eating some items thrice daily, then those items are not food items.

Can a person remain alive just by eating coconut alone? Yes. Then coconut is a food. Can a person remain alive just by smoking cigarettes? No. Then cigarette is an intoxicant. A person can live just by eating non veg. food alone. So, non-veg. items are food. Can a person live just by smoking Ganja? No. Then, it is an intoxicant. Food is an item which carries nutrients from outside into our body. Intoxicant is an item which takes away the nutrients already stored in our body.

Therefore, when we use a narcotic, our body will get more stamina for some specific period of time. After that, we will be without stamina. This is because the narcotic will spend away the nutrients already stored in our body and thus make us less potent. Moreover, narcotics never supply any nutrients to our body. Therefore, we should never consume
narcotics.

Many people say, "I go to the doctor and take treatment for several years. But my disease has not been cured." But, these people never reveal anything about the narcotics they use. Therefore, consuming tea, coffee, etc. is more injurious to our health than eating non-vegetarian food. Please understand about the food types mentioned above and check which of these types you consume.
As far as possible, we should move towards Type 1 foods. Some nature-cure doctors say that we should eat only natural food all three times daily.

This is very hard to follow in practice. If you keep eating only natural food thrice daily continuously for one month, saliva will flow in your tongue when you see your favourite dish. You will be tempted to eat it and you will find it very hard to resist. To solve this problem, we offer you a simple solution. Eat only uncooked foods in the mornings.

Then the pranic energy and minerals needed by your body will be obtained in a natural way through the breakfast. Let the lunch consist of cooked food.

Eat whatever dishes you want to your heart's content during lunch. This is for satisfying your desire for taste. Since we should not eat much during the night, take only rice porridge, wheat porridge or any other porridge along with any cooked vegetable dish for dinner. If you eat in this way, you will be eating natural food and at the same time you will have the satisfaction of eating cooked food as per your desire.

Also, you will be eating porridge which is a medicine that can cure many diseases. Then, nutrients will reach our body in all the ways and it will pave the way for our being healthy forever. There is a proverb: "Breakfast like a king, lunch like a prince and dinner like a pauper!" This is the right way to a healthy life. But, what do we do? In a hurry, we eat very little food for breakfast like a beggar and rush to our office.

We eat lunch in a measured way like a Minister. We eat our dinner like a King by gobbling all sorts of food. Our overeating during dinner is the main reason for our getting diseases. The digestive power of our stomach will be more during morning hours. So, please eat your breakfast to your heart's desire in a calm and contented way. Let the lunch be in
a measured way. Reduce the amount of food intake during dinner as much as possible.

This is because we do less physical work during night time and also there will be no sunlight to help us in digesting the food. Heat is needed for our body to digest. the food. We are active during the day time as we walk, run and do a lot of other works. Thus, our body gets heated up through these physical activities. Moreover, when there is sunlight, heat energy comes into our body naturally. Therefore, we should eat more during daytime and eat less during night hours.

How Much Should We Eat

The quantity of food needed by a person will change based on the quantity of work done by the person, the person's body weight, the person's age, mental stamina, behavioral nature, the climate, the natural circumstances, the country, the locality, the town, etc.

All right, then how to find out how much we should eat? There is an easy method for this. We should eat only when we feel hungry. When we eat, if we focus all our attention on the food, then we will not like to eat beyond a certain quantity. When the same food which was tasty when we put it in our mouth for the first time is not tasty anymore, it is a signal for us to stop eating.

Let us say that you are a person who usually eats six Rotis for breakfast. Start eating by focusing your attention on the Roti and its taste. After eating four Rotis in this manner, when you see the fifth Roti you will not feel like eating it. Once you stop liking to eat it, it means that your quota is over.

When we eat with our attention on the food, we will know the amount of food that we need. But, we are engaged in talking, watching TV or speaking over cell phone, etc. When we do so, we do not know how much we need to eat. Therefore, please observe by eating with your attention on the food and its taste. If we eat in this manner, we cannot eat beyond a limit.

When we get the thought in our mind that we have had enough of it, then we have to stop eating. So, henceforth please eat to your heart's content. There is nothing wrong if you eat a little more. Your next hunger time will be slightly postponed. That is all. There is nothing wrong if you eat a little less. You will feel hungry again a little early. That is all Therefore, please do not measure the food that you eat. Whatever amount is desired by you, eat it to your heart's content. But please remember one important point. You should not eat anything again till you feel hungry again.

5.Environmental conditions

Check whether your environment is as follows, or otherwise change it as below.

- Well ventilated working and living environment
- Peaceful noiseless environment
- Good positive people around yourself, They helps you to thought positively.
- Organic garden in your home. Your can get your own organic food.
- Clean environment.

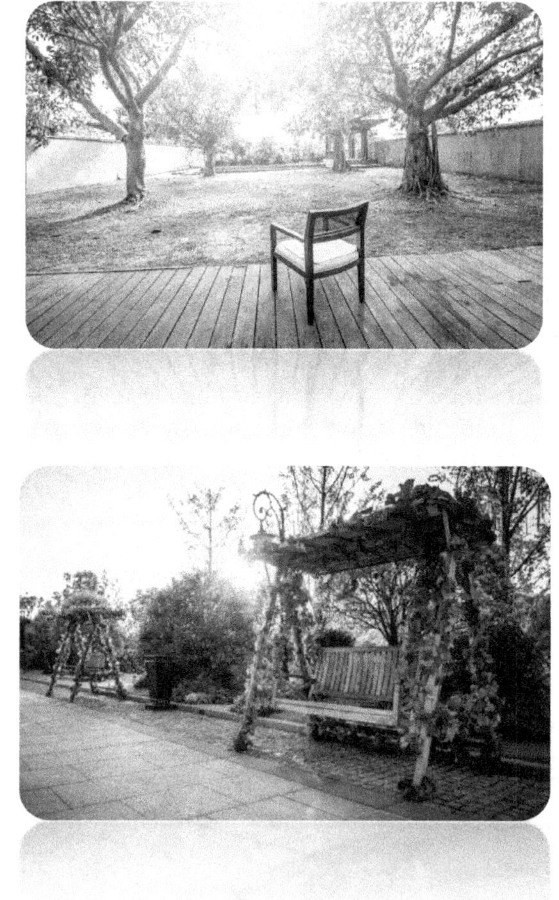

6. Your habits

FOOD HABITS

1. Relation between Eating and Bathing

Many of us have the habit of eating food immediately after taking a bath or a shower. If you eat immediately after taking bath, the food will not be digested properly. We have to eat only after 45 minutes from the time of our finishing the bath. Also, we should take bath only after two and half hours from the time we finish eating food.

The temperature of human body is always 37 degrees Centigrade. Even when we are in a cold climate or a hot climate, the organ called Triple Warmer in our body will always try to keep our body temperature uniformly at 37 degrees Centigrade at all times.

When we take bath, irrespective of whether it is normal water or hot water, irrespective of whether we take bath only for our body excluding the head or including the head, irrespective of whether we take bath in a river, pond or in our bath room, our body temperature will undergo a change immediately.

When our body temperature changes, the temperature controlling organ in our body will start working immediately and it will attempt to bring the body temperature to 37 degrees again. When the body is engaged in this activity to restore the body temperature, the digestive organs in the body will not get energy. On an average, the Triple Warmer in our body works for about 45 minutes after we take bath. During this period, the digestive glands in our body will not function.

Therefore, please do not eat immediately after taking bath. Wait for about 45 minutes after finishing the bath and then eat. Similarly, we should take bath only after a period of two and half hours after eating food. This is because it takes two and half hours for the food we eat to get digested and enter our blood stream. Some people may have their food digested in one hour. It may take up to five hours for some other people. So, we can safely assume that it takes about two and half hours on an average to digest the food.

Let us assume that we take bath within half an hour after eating the food. Immediately after we take bath, the temperature control organ in our body will start acting to set right the temperature of the body. At that time, all the energy in the body will be spent by the temperature control organ and no energy will be available to the digestive organs for performing their duties. You can check this for yourself.

Take bath immediately after eating food just for one day. You will get digestive problem on that day. You will feel uncomfortable in your stomach. You will get headache. Therefore, we should not take bath for a period of two and half hours after eating food. We should wait for a period of 45minutes after taking bath before we start eating food.

2. Taste of Food

Sometimes we feel very tired. If we do not eat food for several hours, our body will be very dull. When we are in a position where we cannot even walk, we may eat some food. Do we get energy in our body immediately after eating the food or few hours later? We get energy immediately after eating the food. But, scientifically, the food we eat through our mouth goes to the stomach and remains there for a few hours and gets digested, then goes to the small intestine and gets digested there for a few hours and then mixes in the blood.

Therefore, we should get energy only after a few hours. Have you noticed that sugar level is tested in the hospitals only when two hours have passed after eating the food? The reason for this is that the food we eat gets converted into sugar and mixes with the blood only after two hours. But we get energy immediately after eating the food. Where does this energy come from? A certain amount of energy is obtained from the tastes in the food that we eat.

Therefore, from now on, by adding all the six tastes namely sweet, salt, pungent, sour, bitter and astringent tastes in every course of food that we eat, we can increase our digestive power and we can convert our food into medicine.

In some countries, people eat only sweet, bitter and astringent tastes in their food and they do not add salt, sour and pungent tastes. In some other countries, such as India, people eat only salt, sour and hot tastes and they do not add sweet, bitter and astringent tastes. Thus, people in different countries eat some tastes and do not eat some tastes. This is the basic reason for diseases. Therefore, we should try to eat food containing all the six tastes in each and every course of food that we eat.

3. Eat Only When You Are Hungry

Just by following this one small guideline we can get the food digested properly. This guideline is that we have to eat only when we are hungry. What is hunger? Hunger is nothing but the signal to us from our body that all the parts in our body are ready for digesting the food properly and mix it with the blood.

All the food that we eat without feeling hungry become waste or poison. One very important secret in our treatment is that we should eat only when we feel hungry. People say that no disease will come if you take food as per a time schedule. This is wrong. Whoever eats food in a timely manner, they will get all the diseases. Eating when you are hungry is totally different from eating timely food.

For example, let us say that we took breakfast at 8.00 am in the morning. Let us assume that we did not give any appreciable work to our body after breakfast. Now we see that the clock shows 2.00 pm. We think, "Oh, it is already 2.00 pm! Let us take lunch."

But did we check whether we feel hungry? No. If you see the time and eat lunch at 2.00 pm when even the breakfast that you ate in the morning is not yet digested and mixed in the blood, you will get diseases. The food in the stomach also will not be digested. The food that you consume now also will not be digested. So, the first reason for all the diseases in the world is eating without feeling hungry.

Let us see another example. You eat your breakfast at 8.00 am in the morning. Then you work hard. You feel hungry at 12.00 noon. What will happen if you wait without taking food saying, "I will not eat now; I will eat food as per time schedule; I will eat only at 2.00 pm"? The hydrochloric acid in the stomach will be secreted by 12.00 noon when you feel hungry. Since this acid does not get any food till 2.00 pm, it will be diluted.

Thus, the food that you eat two hours after you get hunger will not be digested properly. What we have to understand from this is that, if you eat timely food you will get diseases. If you eat food when you are hungry you will not get diseases and the diseases that you may already have will be cured.

Who has invented the law that everyone should eat thrice daily? Some people may do more physical work. They can eat even five times a day. Some people will do less physical work, It may be sufficient if they eat twice a day. Therefore, from now on, please do not see the clock for eating. We have to keep on doing our work. Only when our body creates the feeling of hunger in us, we have to think about eating food and only then we have to eat food.

The great sage Thiruvalluvar says in the immortal Tamil epic Thirukkural, "The body does not need medicine for any disease. After the food that we eat is digested, we

need to eat food when we feel hungry again. If we follow this, then our body will not need any medicine at all for any disease." Thus, one important principle in our treatment is that we have to eat only when we feel hungry. If you do not follow this principle and follow all other principles that we are going to explain after this, then you may not get the best results.

When we eat thrice daily, we eat 90 times in a month. It may not be possible for all of us to eat after feeling hungry at all these 90 times. Therefore, to start with, we can practice eating after feeling hungry for at least 10 times in a month. Then we can increase it to 20, 30 and so on.

Some of us may work in a company. We may be required to eat lunch between 1.00 PM and 2.00 PM and return to work at 2.00 PM. What can we do if we do not feel hungry.

During that time? In this way, there may be a necessity to eat food without feeling hungry sometimes. During such times.   Eat little bit excess or less as suitable for your lunch time. By doing so, we can save ourselves from having our food being converted into waste and poison. However, it is always good to wait for hunger when we are at our home and also wherever we can. So, please eat your food only after you feel hungry.

When we eat food, we should mix it with saliva and eat. Only the food that mixes with the saliva goes to the blood as good food. The food which does not mix with saliva goes to the blood as bad food. Our saliva contains a lot of enzymes. These enzymes help very much in separating the constituents from the food. Only the food that has been digested by the saliva in the mouth can be digested by the stomach. When the food that has not been digested by the saliva goes into the stomach, it becomes bad food and waste matter.

Many of us may say, "We do mix saliva with food when we eat." However, this is not true. Whoever eats food with their lips open when they chew the food, for these people saliva will not mix with the food. When we chew the food, the lips should be closed. Only then the saliva will mix with the food. What is the difference between keeping the lips open and keeping them closed when we chew the food?

Imagine the food as a ball, and saliva as another ball. When we eat with the lips open, the air goes inside the mouth, stands between the saliva and the food and does not allow them to mix. Thus, it prevents proper digestion in the mouth. Air is the enemy to the digestion in the mouth. Therefore, from now on whenever you eat any food, please open your lips only for sending the food inside the mouth.

Once the food is inside the mouth, keep chewing the food without separating the lips till you swallow the food. In countries such as USA, UK, Italy, etc. the prevalence of Diabetes is very less. This is because the people of these countries have the habit of chewing the food with their lips closed.

The people in India, Sri Lanka, Malaysia, Singapore, etc. eat keeping their lips open, the sugar disease is more prevalent in these countries. Please do not immediately conclude that the people of some countries are intelligent and the people of some other countries are foolish. People in some countries consume more medicines for mental illnesses.

Many people in countries having the habit of eating with their lips closed are affected by mental illnesses and consume medicines for these diseases. Thus, in some countries body is not all right but mind is all right. In some other countries, mind is not all right but body is all right. So, the business is running fine for the drug manufacturing companies in all the countries. Therefore, from now on, please chew every mouthful of food keeping your lips closed

5. Keep your Attention On The Food

when we eat our food, only if our focus and attention are on the thought that we are eating, all the glands concerned to digestion will secrete well. Instead, if we think about family, business, children, etc. while eating food, the digestive glands do not secrete and we get diseases. Therefore, please concentrate your attention on the food while eating the food.

While eating, take the food in your hand and eat it with the thought that this food is going to go inside your stomach, get digested and converted into blood, become food for all the body parts and function as medicine for all diseases. Then we can have a healthy life.

The golden rule is, Eat food only when you feel hungry; While eating, think only about food. So please avoid cellphone, tv,books while eating

6. Grind well the food in Your Mouth

When we eat, we should grind it well using our teeth and then swallow it. Whoever swallows their food as it is without breaking and grinding the food with their teeth, their stomach will ask them one question: "Do I have any teeth to grind the food? Or do I have any mixer blades or grinder?" There are no teeth or mixer blades or grinder in the stomach. Then how does the stomach digest the food we eat?

We should chew the food, grind it well using our teeth and then only swallow it. Generally, we do not give much work to our teeth at all. We just swallow the food in big morsels.

Let us assume that we take the food 40 times with our hand when we eat a plate of food. If we eat the food without properly chewing it during the first four times, the acid that is available in the stomach for digesting the 40 handfuls of food will be exhausted after digesting 4 handfuls of food.

This is because the acid in the stomach has to do the job which is supposed to have been done by the teeth. So, only the first four mouthfuls of food become good blood. The next 36 mouthfuls of food become waste and go out as stool because there is no acid in the stomach to digest it. The only reason for pot belly and obesity is that we do not give much work to our teeth.

7. Connection between water & digestion

We should not drink water for half an hour before we start eating our food. We should not drink water in between while eating the food. We should not drink water immediately after we finish eating the food. And, we should not drink water for at least half an hour after we finish eating the food. Some people drink one glass of water and then start eating their food.

These people will not have their food digested properly. It is because of the following reason. We have seen that the hydrochloric acid that is secreted in the stomach is what digests the food. If we drink water just before eating the food, this acid will be diluted. Once this acid is diluted, whatever good food that we may eat and however well we may eat it, it will not be digested
properly.

We should not drink water in between our eating the food. The digestion will be spoiled if we do so. Those who bite and chew the food well, make it a paste, mix it with saliva and then swallow it will not feel like drinking water while eating the food. We should not drink water immediately after finishing the eating. Many of us drink one or two glasses of water immediately after finishing the eating. This also will spoil the digestion. We have to wait for about half an hour after we finish the eating and then only drink water. Thus, half an hour before start of food, half an hour during eating, assuming that we take about half an hour for eating, and half an hour after finishing the food means that we should not drink water for one and a half hour in total. How can we totally avoid drinking water for one and a half hours?

During this period, we may get hiccups, thirst, throat drying up, tongue drying up,food being hot and spicy, etc. Why should we drink water when the food is hot, spicy and pungent? Our tongue tells us, "The food is hot and spicy." That is all. Did it ask us to drink water? No. If the food is hot and spicy, then we have to find ways to reduce the hot taste and we should not drink water.

So, when the food is hot and pungent, we have to mix some coconut oil, sesame oil, etc. with the food and reduce the hot and spicy taste. If some oil goes with the food, even then digestion will be done well. But, if water goes with the food, it will spoil the digestion. Therefore, if the food is spicy, find alternative ways to reduce the taste and avoid drinking water.

What can we do if we get hiccups while eating? First of all, let us see why we get hiccups while eating. A person who focuses his attention on the food while eating will not get hiccups. The Vagus nerve connects our brain and the other parts of the body. While eating, if we have only the thought about the food in our mind, then this nerve will keep all the glands concerned with digestion working well.

Suddenly, if our mind starts thinking about the family, business or any other person, this nerve will get confused. There will be dilemma whether the gland concerned with digestion should secrete or the gland concerned with the emotions we have should secrete. Hiccups occur only due to this confusion.

When people get hiccups, they say that someone is thinking about them at that time. In fact, no one is thinking about you when you have hiccups. On the other hand, you are thinking about someone and that is why you are getting the hiccups. So, as long as you keep thinking about the food while eating, you will not get hiccups.

What should we do if the tongue is dried up or if we feel thirsty? During the one and half hours, if our throat dries up or if we feel thirsty or if we get hiccups, we can drink water. But there is a limit to it.

We should drink less quantity of water so that the water we drink does not reach our stomach. If our throat has dried up, then the water should just wet the throat and if our tongue is dried up, then the water we drink should just wet the tongue.

That is, the water should be so less in quantity that it wets just our lips, mouth, tongue and gullet. The water should not reach the stomach. Thus, we need to understand that air is the enemy for the digestion done in the mouth and water is the enemy for the digestion done in the stomach.

We can just wet our mouth before eating the food using one fourth glass of water so that it does not reach the stomach. While eating the food, if it is very essential that we have to drink water, then we can drink one fourth glass of water so that it does not reach the stomach. Many of us drink nearly one glass or one vessel of water immediately after eating the food. Please do not do this.

After finishing the eating, it is sufficient if we drink one fourth to half glass of water just for gargling the mouth. Then please wait for half an hour. After that, we can drink liberally two glasses of water or even more and it will not cause any harm to the digestion. So, half an hour before starting the food, during the eating and half an hour after finishing the food, avoid drinking water as far as possible. If needed, please drink very limited quantity of water.

Water drinking Habits

8. How much Liter of water per day ..?

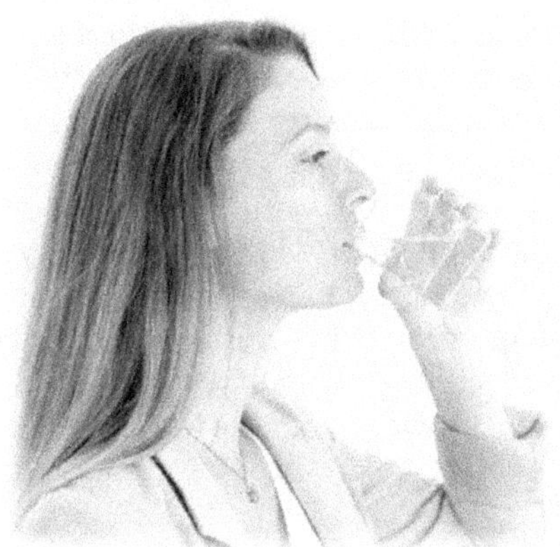

There is no compulsion that a person should drink a specific quantity of water every day. If you drink two litres of water in cold countries such as Switzerland, Norway,etc. your kidney will be damaged within a week. On the other hand, two litres of water daily will not at all be sufficient for the people living in deserts.

A person who is engaged in the job of laying roads from morning to evening under the hot sun on the hot tar, wearing boots and helmet will definitely need more than five litres of water in a day.

However, for a computer engineer who works in the air-conditioned room, one litre per day will be enough.

When a person who works on the road on a particular day travels with his friend in an air-conditioned car the next day his water requirement would change. Thus, nobody can accurately say how much quantity of water a human being should drink in a day. The quantity will vary depending on his age, height, weight, weather, country, his mental state, his work, the rooms or places where he works, air conditioning, etc.

So, we cannot accept that a person should compulsorily drink a specific quantity of water in a day. If someone drink sunder the compulsion that a definite quantity of water should be consumed in a day, his kidney will be overloaded and will get damaged. All right, then how to find out how much quantity of water a person should drink in a day? I do not know. Neither do you. Then who knows? Only your body knows.

So, we should drink water only when we feel thirsty. When you feel thirsty, you should drink as much quantity of water as you like, as per your heart's desire. Then we should forget about water and keep doing our work. When we feel thirsty again, only then we should drink water again. Those people in cold areas will get thirsty about four times in a day. Each time, if they drink a quarter of a litre of water, their thirst will be quenched. In hot areas, people will feel thirsty ten times in a day.

Each time half a litre of water will be required. When a person living in a cold area today goes to a hot area tomorrow, his thirst level will change. So, all the people who drink water under the compulsion that they should drink a specific quantity of water every day are actually drinking water more or less than the actual requirement of their body. This excess or shortage of water causes diseases in their body.

Therefore, please do not measure the water you drink. When you feel thirsty you should drink as much water as required and you should drink water again when you feel thirsty again, to the extent of requirement. If you do so, your body will inform you how much water is needed today and it will receive that much water. This is the right quantity of water that we should drink everyday

9. We Should Consume water Slowly Sipping It.

we should slowly sip the water and eat it as though it is a solid. Water contains all the six tastes. By slowly sipping the water, we can get all the six tastes that are needed by our body from the water we drink. When water is mixed with the saliva and then the water goes inside, our body gets a lot of benefits. Moreover, a part called tonsil in our body helps to remove the germs from the water and also to bring the water to our body temperature.

Those who drink water in one go by directly pouring water into their throat are likely to get diseases in their tonsils. This is because, when water goes very fast past the tonsil, the tonsil is forced to do its job very fast. So, there is a possibility of the tonsil getting diseases. The slower we drink water our body will get better health and more power. Then we will not get problems with tonsil and diseases related to breathing such as wheezing, chest cold, sinus, etc. Even if we get any such disease, it will be cured immediately. So, we should drink water by slowly sipping it and enjoying its taste.

10. Drink Water Immediately After Passing Urine.

Whenever we pass urine, it means that we need water at that time. So, our body will be healthy if we drink at least a small quantity of water after passing urine. Therefore, if possible, let us drink a small quantity of water after we pass urine.

Sleep

11. Understand the Sleep And Rest

Generally all the doctors say that a person should compulsorily sleep for at least eight hours in a day. But, there is no need to measure the duration of our sleep. We normally do three types of work. The first is the work related to the body. The second is the work related to the mind. The third is the work related to the brain.

Let us see which of these works are related to the sleep. Some people give more work only for their body. They may not give much work to their mind and brain. These people belong to the first category. Those who do physical labour are examples of this category. It does not mean that these people do not use their brains at all. They do not give as much work to their mind and brain as they give to their body.

Therefore, sleep is needed only when you give work to your body. Only then you will get sleep. Sleep is not required when you give work to your mind and brain. So, if you do not get sleep immediately after going to the bed, please do not get agitated and perturbed about it. We will get sleep only when sleep is needed for us. Why should we expect to sleep when it is not needed? Why should we be worried about it?

Thus, we should sleep on our own when we lie down. We should wake up on our own from our bed. If we sleep and wake up in this way, it will be a proper, healthy, peaceful and satisfactory sleep. But many of us are worried if we do not get sleep when we go to the bed. We think, "The BP may be high. The sugar may be low. Or we may have some other disease." We thus unnecessarily imagine many things, needlessly fear and further entangle our mind and brain. If we lie down worrying about not getting sleep, this is a very big disease by itself. Thus, if we have fear, get mentally affected and lie in the bed, our sleep is further delayed.

This is because we confuse our mind and brain more and more. So, more time is needed to sort out these worries and concerns also. If you do not get sleep one day, there is no need to sleep on that day. If you do not get sleep for one or two days, do not worry about it. You will sleep sufficiently on the third day to cover for the three days. Your body has intelligence. It will definitely ask for whatever it needs and get it from us.

12. Don't wake Up with Alarm

Many of us have the habit of waking up to the sound of the alarm clock. When we are in deep sleep in the morning, when our entire body is sleeping peacefully and calmly, suddenly we are forced to wake up when the alarm clock sounds loud. If our sleep is interrupted by the alarm clock in this way, our body gets affected it gets a kind of tension. This tension will prevail in us throughout that day.

Therefore, please do not use the alarm clock to wake up Just think. What would have happened if the alarm clock had not sounded? We would have slept for about two m o r e h o u r s . What does this mean ?

This means that our body needs two more hours of sleep. When our body needs more sleep, if we cut it short and wake up who will make up for that sleep? If we wake up every day using alarm clock and cut two or three hours of our sleeping time,after some time, we might be forced to go into sleep forever. So, please do not use the alarm clock.

Some people may ask, "We have to get up early. How can we get up without using an alarm clock?" We get and give lot of advice that we have to get up early in the morning. But nobody advises that we have to go to bed early every night. We can get up early in the morning only if we go to the bed early in the night. It is our mistake to do unnecessary things such as watching television, movies, etc. up to 1.00 am or 2.00 am in the night and then go to bed late. Why do you think that even if a person goes to bed at 2.00 am in the night he should get up early in the morning?

If a person goes to bed late he has to get up from the bed late only. According to the time by which we have to get up in the morning, we have to go to bed about 8 hours in advance. Therefore, we have to understand that using an alarm clock is dangerous and we should use the alarm clock only occasionally, that too only for emergency purposes and not on a daily basis. There is a simple solution for those who have a lot of confusion in their mind and do not get sleep for a long time in the night.

Rest will be obtained only in a slow manner if we lie down and rest. But, if we sit and take rest, we will get rest fast. Those who donot get sleep immediately after going to bed can try to sleep by sitting instead of lying down fully, by being in a slanting position, giving some support to our back and our head, closing the eyes, calmly stretching the legs or folding the legs in a squatting position. If we sleep in a sitting posture, our mind and brain sort themselves out very quickly and we will immediately get sleep.

13. Avoid over consuming of Tea, Coffee

Tea, coffee and all the intoxicants are enemies to sleep. Those who smoke, consume alcoholic drinks and use other narcotic drugs will not get proper sleep. Unless these people stop using these things they will not getting peaceful sleep. They will also not get good health. Because we already know very well that these alcoholic items and narcotic drugs create damage to the body, we do not want to describe them elaborately here. Now we will see how our sleep will be affected even if we drink tea and coffee.

The chemicals called serotonin and dopamine need to be secreted in the area of our brain for us to get sleep. We will get sleep only if these chemicals are secreted. So, if you have the habit of drinking 5 cups of tea in a day, you will definitely have a problem with your sleep. Therefore, those who worry about their sleep should first come out of their habit of tea, coffee and other intoxicants.

Then definitely you will get good sleep. Tea and coffee should be consumed only by the people who live in the areas where these plants grow. For example, tea plants grow only in cold areas. If we drink tea and coffee in cold areas, we will not get diseases in the body. This is because in cold areas, the body will not have sufficient heat inside and we will feel sluggish and lazy. We may not feel like doing any work. If we drink tea or coffee at that time, the bitter and astringent taste in them and also the ingredients in them instigate our body and make the body work fast.

Thus, there is nothing wrong if tea and coffee are consumed by the people living in the areas where these plants grow. But if we consume them in places where they do not grow, they create disease in the body. In China, people take coffee and tea without milk and in less quantity. They consume it for indigestion. We can also drink, if needed, one fourth glass of tea or coffee without adding milk and without adding white sugar. If we take just two sips it is medicine. But if we take one glass it is poison. Whichever food variety such as vegetables, fruits, etc, grows more in your area, consider them as the food which will improve your health. In some countries rice grows more. In some other countries wheat grows more.

What we have to understand is that the people of the countries where rice grows more will be healthy if they eat rice. The people of the countries where wheat grows more will be healthy if they eat wheat. But we pay high price to buy and eat apple, plums, etc. which are grown more in cold areas and are brought to other towns with much effort and cost. The people in cold areas cannot eat hard items that are eaten by people in hot areas. If they eat them it will not be digested properly.

That is why food items suitable for them grow more there. These items will suit the people who live there but they are not needed for people of other areas. If the people of other areas want, they can eat them just for satisfying their desire, once in a while. But, there is no need to buy them at a high price and eat them.

14. *Don't* lie down with our head in the north direction

What is present in the universe is also present in the body" says a proverb. All the powers in the universe are present in our body also. This includes magnetic power also. Our body functions like a magnet with the upper part above the naval as North Pole and the lower part below the naval as South Pole. North poles of two magnets will repel each other. We cannot bring them together. But opposite poles of two magnets attract each other. If we lie down with our head in the north direction, the north pole of our body and the north pole of the earth's magnet do not attract each other and they repel each other.

Thus, the magnetic repelling action keeps happening throughout the night. So, we cannot sleep peacefully. Our blood circulation will not be properly streamlined. As a result, we will get diseases in the body. Therefore, we should not lie down with our head in the north direction. If we lie down with our head in the south direction, our body's North Pole and the South Pole of the earth will attract each other. Then, we will get peaceful sleep. So, it is a very good idea to sleep with our head in the south direction.

During pregnancy, when the child is in the womb, the mother's magnetic power will have its North Pole in the north direction above the naval and its South Pole will be in the south direction below the naval. But, the child will have its upper part above its naval in the north and its lower part below its naval in the south. Only then the child's head can be facing up. During the tenth month of pregnancy just before the child comes out, a change will happen in this magnetic orientation.

That is, the portion of the child's body above its naval will become its North Pole and the child's body below its naval will become its South Pole. Immediately when this change happens, the child's upper part which is the northern part will turn towards the mother's leg side which is her southern part. This is called the "turning of the child's head". Therefore, please do not lie down with your head in the north direction. It is best to lie down with your head in the southern direction.

15. Brush at Night

Those who worry that they do not get good sleep in the night will get good sleep if they brush their teeth 30 minutes after eating their dinner and then go to bed. But we should not consume anything such as milk or any other items after brushing our teeth. We can drink water if needed. In case we eat some food, then we must brush our teeth again. Thus, as far as sleep is concerned, we should lie down whenever we feel sleepy.

But we should not think that sleep should come immediately when we lie down. Our body will sleep on its own. And it will wake up on its own. In this way, if we give to our body whatever duration of sleep it desires to have, our body gets all the space-related energy in a proper way and it cures all the diseases.

16. Work or activities to body

Heart is the organ in our body which pumps up the blood circulation. Irrespective of whether we think about it or not, whether we remember or not, the heart keeps on doing its work. Similar to the blood circulation system, there is one more system called Lymphatic system in our body. Nobody talks about this and nobody bothers about this system. The blood circulation system is the one which takes the food to all the parts in our body. At the same time, the lymphatic system is the one which takes the medicines to cure diseases to all the parts in our body.

Just like the blood circulation, this lymph also should be always flowing in our body.
But, there is no organ like heart to pump up the lymph circulation in our body. Only those who have physical activity in their body will have this lymph circulation going on in their body. If there is no physical activity, lymph circulation will slow down.

For all the people who have some physical movements, that is, for all those who give work to their body, lymph circulation will be going on. For those who do not give work to their body and are sluggish and lazy, this lymph circulation will not be proper. This is the reason for the occurrence of many diseases. Moreover, diseases which occur do not get cured. This is why we observe that our diseases get cured when we go for walking, do physical exercises, do yoga asanas, etc. Therefore, every person should always be giving some movement, vibration or work to all the muscles and joints in his body every day.

Only then the lymph will run properly and cure all the diseases in the body.

This is why those who do physical work do not get many diseases and those who do not do much physical work get more diseases. Many people come to me and say, "I have a disease for several years. But it is not getting cured even though I have taken many treatments for it." The first question I ask them is, "Do you do any yoga exercise?" many of them reply, "I do not practise Yoga. I do not have time for all that. I tell them, "I am healthy. I do not have any disease. But I am doing some exercise or other every day. When I am healthy and still I am doing some exercise for one or two hours every day, why can't you do yoga exercises when you have a disease already?" Yoga is taught in every town, in every locality nowadays. We can easily learn Yoga and get benefit. If we devote at least half an hour every day for our body and do some exercises, lymph circulation will run properly in our body and we can cure the diseases by ourselves. Many people have a fear about yoga.

They think, "We have to fold and stretch our hands and legs. We have to bend and straighten our back. Can we do all this?" This doubt is present in the minds of many people. Please understand that yoga is not just about folding and stretching our hands and legs. Yoga is an art which integrates and unifies our body, mind, breath, brain and our life. Yoga Asana which consists of folding and stretching our hands and legs is just one part of Yoga. Asanas alone do not constitute Yoga. Yoga consists of totally eight parts.

These are: (1) Iyamam (2) Niyamam (3) A s a n a m (4) P r a n a y a m a m (5)Prathyaakaaram (6) Dhaaranai (7) Dhyaanam (8) Samaadhi.

(1) **IYAMAM**
Iyamam is the art of understanding the things that we should not do. Iyamam is nothing but knowing what are the bad habits and practices followed by us that affect our mind, brain and life and refraining ourselves from doing such things.

(2)**NIYAMAM**
Niyamam is the art of understanding the things that we should do, what are the good habits and practices and what are the benefits of doing these things.

(3) **ASANAM**

Asanam is the exercise by which we give movement to all the muscles, limbs and all the parts of our body and set right the lymph circulation in our body. But many people wrongly understand that yoga means yoga asana.

(4) **PRANAYAMAM**

Our body consists of a Pranic body in it. Pranayama is the art of setting right our Pranic body by streamlining the air that we breathe through several breathing exercises. such as Nadi Suddhi , B a s t h r i k a , Kapaalapathi, Pranayamam, Agnisar, etc.

(5) **PRATHYAAKAARAM**

Prathyaakaaram is the state by which we control or forget the five senses of our body namely seeing, smelling, hearing tasting and touching.

(6) **DHAARANAI**

If our mind keeps on thinking about only one thing, it is called Dhaaranai. Our mind will be contained and controlled if it is thinking only about one thing, say, a flower, our Family God or Goddess or a person whom we like and not thinking about anything else. This state is called Dhaaranai.

(7) **DHYAANAM or Medidation**

What is Dhyaanam? In Dhaaranai, we keep on thinking about only one thing. If we stop thinking even that one thing and we are in a state where we are not thinking about anything and we are simply present without seeing, smelling, listening, tasting, touching and sensing anything at all, this state is called Dhyaanam.

(8) **SAMAADHI**

If we are not thinking about anything for a very short duration such as one or two minutes, this state is called Dhyaanam. If we are in Dhyaanam for a long duration such as one or two hours, then this state is called Samaadhi.

1. FOOD (EARTH)

- We should do a prayer before we start eating the food.
- We should not eat when we are not hungry. We should eat only when we are hungry.
- Our food should contain all the six tastes.
- We should start by eating the sweet taste.
- We should swallow the food only after fully enjoying its taste using our tongue.
- We should chew the food till the tongue stops enjoying all the six tastes.
- When we eat the food, we should close our eyes, chew the food without opening our lips till the food becomes a paste and then swallow it.
- We should not drink water for half an hour before we start eating our food.
- We should not drink water while eating food.
- We should not drink water for half an hour after we finish eating our food.
- Just before we start eating our food and just after we finish eating our food, we should drink a little water by sucking it from our palm.
- We should eat our food only after a gap of 45 minutes after we finish taking bath or shower.
- We should not take bath or shower for a period of 2 and 1/2 hours after we finish eating the food.
- We should not keep talking while we eat our food.

- We should not keep our legs hanging while we eat our food.

- Mother should not sit and eat her food along with her children.

- We should not keep reading any book while we eat our food.

- As far as possible, we should eat food prepared by those who have concern for us.

- While eating we should focus our attention only on the food. We should not think about our business, family, etc. while eating the food.

- Those not having teeth should make the food into a paste using grinder, mixer, etc. and then eat it.

2. DRINKING WATER

- We should drink water by slowly sipping it little by little.

- We should drink water immediately after we pass urine.

- We can filter the water using a cotton cloth and then drink it.

- We can put a banana skin, copper coin or copper plate inside the water for half an hour and then drink the water.

- We can keep water in an earthen pot for two hours and then use it.

- We should clean our drinking water tank frequently.

- We should not use mineral water sold in bottles.

- We should not filter the water using water filter or water purifier.

- We should not drink water when we are not feeling thirsty.

- We should not drink water pouring it into our mouth from above.

- There is no prescribed quantity of water that we have to compulsorily drink every day.

3. AIR

- We should not use mosquito coil, mosquito repellent liquid, mosquito mat, etc.
- There should be good air ventilation at all places such as our home, office, factory, bed room, etc, at all times.
- We should not keep all the windows closed in our bed room when we sleep.
- Use mosquito net to protect yourself from mosquito.
- Air ventilation in the places where we live should be such that good air can come in and bad air can go out for all the 24 hours of the day.

4. REST – SLEEP

- We should not lie down to sleep with our head in the north direction.
- We should not drink tea and coffee.
- We should not lie down on barren floor.
- Those who do physical work should sleep for at least 6 hours everyday. Those who give work to their mind and brain should take rest for at least 6 hours every day.
- We should know the difference between sleep and rest.
- If we brush our teeth before going to bed, we will get good sleep.
- If we massage the area below our jaw, we will get good sleep.
- If we massage between the crown of our head and the top of the head, we will get good sleep.

5. WORK

- We should eat only when we feel hungry.

- The body temperature of a healthy human being is 37 degree Centigrade (98.4 degree Fahrenheit). Therefore, we should adjust the room temperature maintained by the Air Conditioning unit according to the climatic conditions.

- We should eat according to the quantity of work we do or we should do work according to the amount of food we eat.

- We should give work to all the joints in our body every day. Air ventilation in the places where we live But, only our physical work will make our lymph flow. Lymph flow will not be all Our heart helps in making our blood flow. right for those who do not do sufficient physical work. This is the cause of many diseases.

.

Follow the all habits and understand the facts which are explained above, think and compare with the symptoms of your body. Live healthy life. If you are taking medical treatment, don't leave it immediately, follow the above habits and slowly monitor your progress in your health, then you can reduce your medicines.

Send your comments and feedbacks to thiruvalluva15100@gmail.com. These methods and habits were followed by old Indian Tamil people. I would like to thank my guru Mr. Healer Basker who gathering lot of good information from all over the world and teaching to the world as free. I have explained about the diseases and remedies in Vol.2.

Thank you for Reading this book…!

Live a healthy and happy life……!

Prakash. M